IMPERVIOUS HERBS

The most promising herbal compounds for antiviral drug development

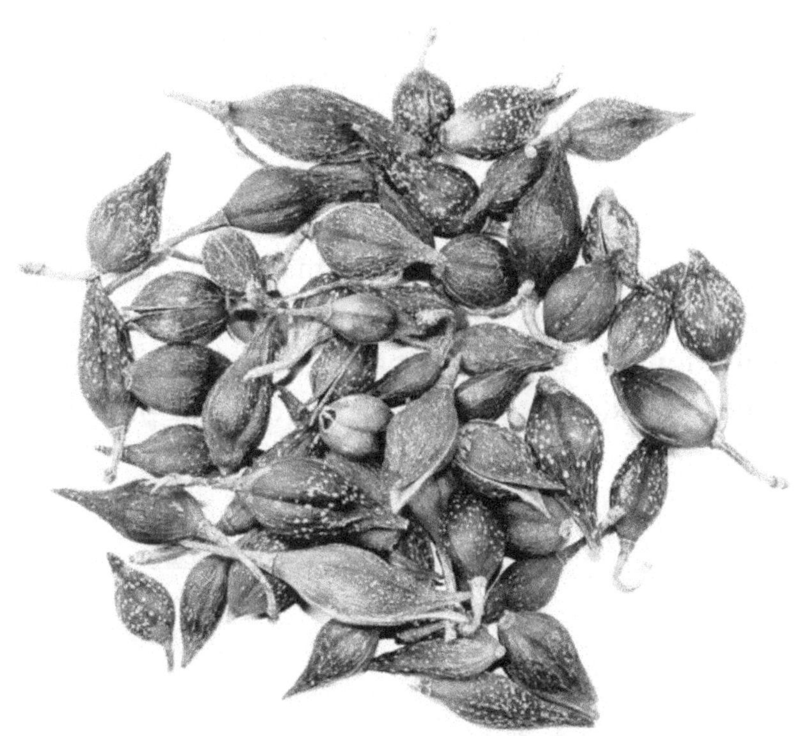

BY ANNE ANGELONE, MS., L.AC.

Table of Contents

Introduction

While herbs in the Traditional Chinese Medicine (TCM) pharmacy offer a treasure trove of potent compounds for viral respiratory infections, we still do not have randomized controlled trials to affirm the most effective ones for the current pandemic. However, the bioactive compounds in herbs and formulas used for other viral respiratory infections, including SARS-CoV-1, have already been thoroughly investigated. In *Functional Herbal Medicine and Phytonutrition*, we reviewed the potent compounds in traditional and empirical formulas now being recommended for SARS-CoV-2. In this guide, we will consider a novel antiviral formula based on current herb and drug development research.

A Novel Antiviral Formula

San Da Jie Du Tang - Three-Hit Resolve Toxins Decoction

In the search for the best antiviral therapeutics, researchers are considering compounds in medicinal herbs that show antiviral activity in terms of blocking SARS-CoV-2 entry and interrupting replication. The current research suggests that potent compounds in herbs, such as flavonoids, terpenoids, and saponins used for SARS-CoV-1, may also have synergistic therapeutic effects against SAR-CoV-2.

In the herbs that contain them, these potent compounds help protect against ultraviolet radiation, microbial infections, and meandering herbivores. These same compounds also confer protective benefits in human beings, as evidenced in an ever-increasing body of research, including animal models and human studies. In a sense, these potent compounds allow these herbs to be somewhat impervious to triggers from the external environment. In this guide, the theme is that these plant compounds also confer a protective (impervious) effect for humans against viral respiratory infections.

All of these compounds regulate a wide range of signaling pathways, such as NFKB and cytokines, which is necessary to modulate the cytokine storm in cases of viral respiratory distress. Combining these compounds in herbal formulas provides a three-hit antiviral, immune-modulating, and anti-inflammatory effect to help decrease the severity of infections, modulate immune activity, and reduce inflammation. For the current pandemic, it is the combination of these synergistic compounds (in herbal formulas) that may all function together to block or inhibit SARS-CoV-2, decrease NFKB and cytokines, and mitigate inflammation. Knowing how to configure them wisely may help propel us through this pandemic.

Given the current research regarding antiviral drug development from natural compounds, a formula to use immediately for initial symptoms of fever, fatigue, and dry cough, should be a combination of potent herbal ingredients that dismantle the virus while also providing respiratory support, immune-modulation, and anti-inflammatory effects. This formula can be called *San Da Jie Du Tang*, which translates as the 'Three-Hit Resolve Toxins Decoction' for its' three-hit antiviral, immune-modulating and anti-inflammatory effects.

In this guide, we will start by reviewing the herbs in the novel antiviral formula *San Da Jie Du Tang* and analyzing how each of the compounds may block entry and replication of SARS-CoV-2. The following chart lists all of the herbs in the novel anti-SARS-CoV-2 formula, *San Da Jie Du Tang.*

San Da Jie Du Tang - Ingredients and Dosages

- Lian Qiao (Fructus Forsythiae) 15g
- Jin Yin Hua (Flos Lonicerae Japonicae) 15g
- Xiang Ru (Herba Moslae) 6g
- Bo He (Herba Menthae Haplocalyx) 9g
- Zi Hua Di Ding (Herba Violae) 9g
- Xiang Chun Ye (Toona Sinensis Roem) 9g
- Sang Ye (Folium Mori) 12g
- Ku Xing Ren (Semen Armeniacae Amarum) 9g
- Ban Lan Gen (Isatis Indigotica) 12g
- Mian Ma Guan Zhong (Dryopteris Crassirhizoma) 9g
- Andrographis Paniculata (Chuan Xin Lian) 6g
- Huang Qin (Scutellaria Baicalensis) 9g
- Da Huang (Rheum Palmatum) 3g
- Wu Bei Zi (Galla Chinensis) 6g
- Yu Xing Cao (Houttuynia Cordata) 15g
- Jie Geng (Radix Platycodi) 6g
- Zhi Shi (Fructus Aurantii Immaturus) 9g
- Huo Xiang (Herba Agastaches Pogostemonis) 12g
- Chen Pi (Pericarpium Citri Reticulatae) 9g
- Gan Cao (Glycyrrhiza Glabra) 9g

The following chart describes the many bioactive compounds and their actions in *San Da Jie Du Tang*. Please note additional studies for each herb referenced in the chart below.

San Da Jie Du Tang Ingredients, Bioactive Compounds, and Actions		
Ingredients	**Herb Name**	**Bioactive Compounds and Actions**
	Jin Yin Hua (Flos Lonicerae Japonicae)	Flos Lonicerae Japonicae could act on the S-protein binding site of the ACE2 receptor to block viral entry of SARS-CoV-2 (Niu et al., 2020; Chan et al., 2020). Luteolin, kaempferol, quercetin, apigenin, rutin, caffeic acid, chlorogenic acid, lonicerin (Xu et al., 2019). Chlorogenic acid in Flos Lonicerae Japonicae has antiviral activity against influenza A (H1N1/H3N2) and inhibition of neuraminidase (Ding et al., 2017).

		Homosecoiridoid alkaloids in Flos Lonicerae Japonicae have antiviral activity against the influenza virus H3N2 (Yu et al., 2013).
	Lian Qiao (Fructus Forsythiae)	Fructus Forsythiae could act on the S-protein binding site of ACE2 to block viral entry of SARS-CoV-2 (Niu et al., 2020; Chan et al., 2020). Fructus Forsythiae contains luteolin, quercetin, kaempferol, rutin, baicalin, wogonin. Lignans (forsythin) triterpenoids (betulinic acid, oleanolic acid, ursolic acid) (Dong et al., 2017). Forsythoside A has antiviral effects against influenza (Law et al., 2017).

	Xing Ren (Semen Armeniacae Amarum)	Amygdalin inhibits NFKB and NLRP3 signaling pathways in LPS-induced acute lung injury (Zhang et al., 2017). Amygdalin has an antitussive effect (Miyagoshi et al., 1986).
	Huang Qin (Scutellaria Baicalensis)	Huang Qin (Scutellaria Baicalensis) Baicalin, chrysin, wogonin, and oroxylin A have therapeutic efficacy against acute lung injury caused by influenza A virus (H1N1) (Zhi et al., 2019). Baicalin may have strong binding to the ACE2 enzyme of SARS-CoV-2 (Chen & Du, 2020). Chrysin may inhibit 3CL[pro] and baicalin may inhibit PL[pro] (Wu et al., 2020).

		Scutellarein inhibits the helicase protein of SARS-CoV-1 (Yu et al., 2012). Scutellarin is predicted to bind to the ACE2 receptor to prevent SARS-CoV-2 entry (Chen & Du, 2020). Scutellarin suppresses NLP3 inflammasome activation in macrophages, decreases NFKB, IL-6, TNF-α, and IL-1β (Liu et al., 2018; Wang et al., 2016; Tan et al., 2009). Scutellarin also protects against LPS induced acute lung injury via inhibition of NFKB activation in mice (Tan et al., 2009).

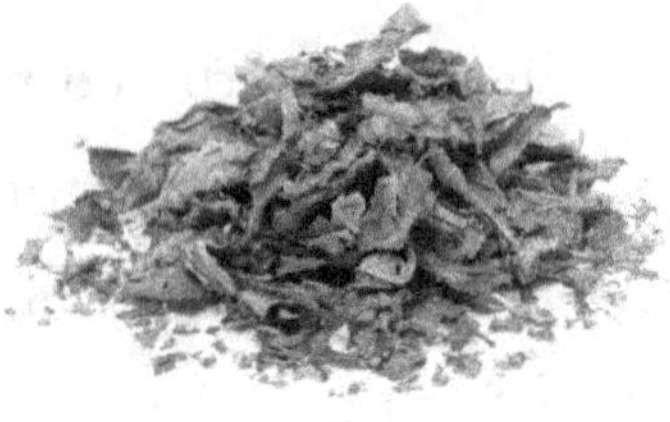	Bo He (Herba Menthae Haplocalyx)	Contains quercetin, apigenin, hesperetin, hesperidin (Zhu, 1998). Diosmin downregulates the expression of T cell receptors, proinflammatory cytokines and NFKB activation against LPS-induced acute lung injury in mice (Imam et al., 2015).
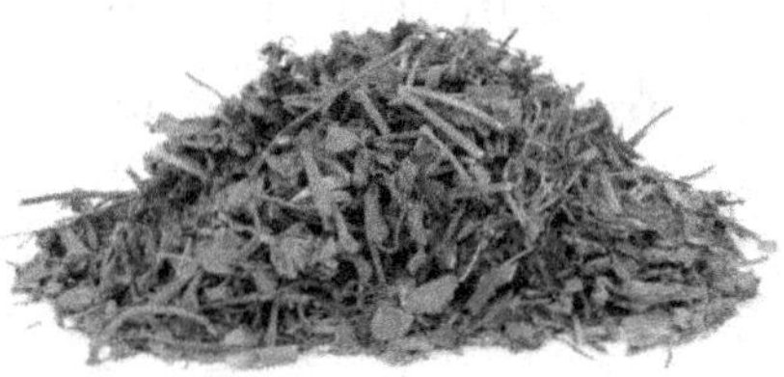	Yu Xing Cao (Houttuynia Cordata)	Houttuynia Cordata (Yu Xing Cao) blocked viral RNA-dependent RNA polymerase activity of SARS-CoV-1 (Lau et al., 2008). Quercetin, quercetrin, and cinanserin from the water extract of Houttuynia Cordata (Yu Xing Cao) inhibits SARS-CoV-1 3CL^{pro} (Lau et al., 2008). Plant polysaccharides from Houttuynia Cordata (Yu Xing Cao) were shown to reduce pulmonary edema,

		protein exudation, and the deposition of complement activation products, thereby mitigating acute lung injury in rats (Lu et al., 2018).
	Ban Lan Gen (Isatis Indigotica)	Sinigrin, β-sitosterol, and indigo dose-dependently inhibited cleavage activities of the $3CL^{pro}$ (Lin et al., 2015). Phaitanthrin D and 2,2-di (3-indolyl)-3-indolone from *Isatis Indigotica* (Ban Lan Gen) may inhibit PL^{pro} (Wu et al., 2020).
	Toona Sinensis Roem (Xiang Chun Ye)	Toona Sinensis Roem (Xiang Chun Ye) contains quercetin, gallic acid, kaempferol, rutin, catechin, epicatechin, β-sitosterol, toosendanin, and phytol (Chia et al., 2007). Quercetin demonstrates potential for M^{pro} inhibition of SARS-CoV-2 (Khaerunnisa et al., 2020).

		TSL-1 extracted from Toona Sinensis Roem (Xiang Chun Ye) inhibits replication of SARS-CoV-1 (Chen et al., 2008).
	Gan Cao (Radix Glycyrrhizae)	Glycyrrhiza Glabra contains the antiviral triterpenoid saponin, glycyrrhizin, found to inhibit SARS-CoV-1 (Cinatl et al., 2003). Glycyrrhizin is predicted to bind to the ACE2 receptor to prevent SARS-CoV-2 entry (Chen & Du, 2020). Glycyrrhizin inhibits IL-6 in macrophages (Liu et al., 2014). Isoliquiritigenin inhibits NFKB activation to suppress the inflammatory response in ARDS (Lago et al., 2014).

	Da Huang (Rheum Palmatum)	Emodin from genus Rheum Palmatum (Da Huang) blocks 3CL[pro] (Luo et al., 2009) and markedly inhibited the interaction of SARS-CoV-1 S-protein and ACE2 (Ho et al., 2007). Emodin inhibits the 3a (viral) ion channel of SARS-CoV-1 and may potentially prevent viral release from infected cells (Schwarz et al., 2011; Schwarz et al., 2014).
	Huo Xiang (Giant Hyssop, Agastaches)	Patchouli alcohol contained in Guang Huo Xiang (Herba Pogostemonis) inhibits 3CL[pro] and, therefore, viral replication of SARS-CoV-2 (Wu et al., 2020). Patchouli alcohol in Guang Huo Xiang (Herba Pogostemonis) also acts on the ACE2 receptor to prevent viral entry (Wu et al., 2020).

		Contains pachypodol, a tri-O-methyl ether of quercetin that inhibits several human pathogenic RNA viruses, including rhinovirus, coxsackievirus and poliovirus, acting on viral plus-strand RNA replication (Ishitsuka et al., 1982).
	Xiang Ru (Herba Moslae)	Herba Moslae (Xiang Ru) contains many similar flavonoids as Herba Ephedrae (Ma Huang), including luteolin, quercetin, and apigenin (Hu et al., 2010). Huang Lian Xiang Ru Decoction has significant effects on H1N1 influenza by enhancing the body's antioxidant capacity, regulating the body's immune function and the host's TLRs pathway (Wu et al., 2016).

	Mian Ma Guan Zhong (Dryopteris Crassirhizoma)	Mian Ma Guan Zhong contains kaempferol, which blocks PL^{pro} and $3CL^{pro}$, and has the potential to inhibit SARS-CoV-2 (Zhang et al., 2020).
	Zhi Shi (Fructus Aurantii Immaturus)	Hesperidin and neohesperidin demonstrate potential as M^{pro} inhibitors (Khaerunnisa et al., 2020). Hesperetin is predicted to bind to the ACE2 receptor to prevent SARS-CoV-2 entry (Chen & Du, 2020). Hesperidin has high binding affinity to the helicase protein of SARS-CoV-2 (Wu et al., 2020). Hesperidin ameliorates acute lung injury (ALI) by inhibiting HMGB1 release (Liu et al., 2015).

		Fructus Aurantii Immaturus contains hesperidin, neohesperidin, hesperetin, rutin, rhoifolin, naringin (Bai et al., 2018). Naringin has a protective effect against ALI (Fouad et al., 2016).
	Chen Pi (Pericarpium Citri Reticulatae)	Nobiletin ameliorates inflammation in acute lung injury by suppression of NFKB pathway in vivo and vitro (Li et al., 2018). Hesperetin from Pericarpium Citri Reticulatae is predicted to bind with ACE2 (Chen & Du, 2020).
	Jie Geng (Radix Platycodi)	Saponin, platycodin D, attenuates acute lung injury by suppressing apoptosis and inflammation in vivo and in vitro (Tao et al., 2015). Platycodin D demonstrated high binding affinity to PL^{pro} (Wu et al., 2020).

	Wu Bei Zi (Galla Chinensis)	Tetra-O-galloyl-β-D-glucose (TGG) from Galla Chinensis (Wu Bei Zi) has been shown to bind with the surface spike (S2) protein of SARS-CoV-1 to block entry into the host cell (Yi et al., 2004).
	Folium Mori (Sang Ye)	Flavonoids: Rutin, isoquercitrin, astragalin, kaempferol, quercetin, chlorogenic acid (Zhang et al., 2017). Quercetin, kaempferol, rutin, morin (Chen et al., 2018). Rutin, isoquercitrin, astragalin, gallic acid (Kim et al., 2014).
	Andrographis Paniculata (Chuan Xin Lian)	Andrographolide is predicted to inhibit 3CL^{pro} and helicase proteins of SARS-CoV-2 (Wu et al., 2020).

		Neoandrographolide in Andrographis Paniculata (Chuan Xin Lian) demonstrated potential for TMPRSS2 inhibition (Wu et al., 2020). Andrographis Paniculata contains andrographolide, neoandrographolide, apigenin, luteolin (Rafi et al., 2020).
	Viola Diffusa (Zi Hua Di Ding)	2β-hydroxy-3,4-seco-friedelolactone-27-oic acid, isodecortinol, and cerevisterol from Viola Diffusa demonstrate potential as 3CL[pro] inhibitors (Wu et al., 2020). Viola Diffusa also contains luteolin, quercetin and anthocyanin.

Analysis of San Da Jie Du Tang - Three-Hit Resolve Toxins Decoction

The coronavirus encodes many proteins, including the most well studied main protease, M^{pro}, (also known as 3C-like protease ($3CL^{pro}$), papain-like protease (PL^{pro}), and the Spike (S)-protein. For herbs to be considered effective antivirals against SARS-CoV-2, they must interfere with the viral attachment, entry, and replication process. A novel antiviral herbal formula would ideally act on all levels to inhibit the damaging effects of SARS-CoV-2.

This includes ACE2 blockade, $3CL^{pro}/M^{pro}$inhibition, PL^{pro} inhibition, Spike protein binding, helicase inhibition, RNA- dependent RNA polymerase (RdRp) inhibition, viroporin 3a ion channel inhibition, and TMPRSS2 inhibition. Let's briefly review the herbs and compounds that have been studied for each of these effects. Please read through each section to identify the herb compounds that inhibit these enzymes and, therefore, viral attachment and replication.

1. ACE2 Blockade

Researchers have started considering that the same active plant compounds, which blocked ACE2 of SARS-CoV-1, might also prevent SARS-CoV-2 from attaching to ACE2. The most studied compounds that demonstrated the potential to interact with and block ACE2 include glycyrrhizin, scutellarin, hesperetin, emodin, chlorogenic acid, forsythoside A, and patchouli alcohol (Cinatl et al., 2007; Ho et al., 2007; Chen and Du, 2020; Niu et al., 2020; Wu et al., 2020).

The herbs that contain these compounds include Gan Cao (Radix Glycyrrhizae), Huang Qin (Scutellaria Baicalensis), Chen Pi (Pericarpium Citri Reticulatae), Da Huang (Rheum Palmatum), Jin Yin Hua (Flos Lonicerae Japonicae), Lian Qiao (Fructus Forsythiae), and Huo Xiang (Herba Agastaches Pogostemonis).

The following chart lists the herbs and compounds in *San Da Jie Du Tang* that might target ACE2. Please note additional studies for each herb referenced in the chart below.

Compounds in San Da Jie Du Tang That Might Target ACE2		
Ingredients	Herb Name	Bioactive Compounds and Actions
	Jin Yin Hua (Flos Lonicerae Japonicae)	Flos Lonicerae Japonicae could act on the S-protein binding site of the ACE2 receptor to block viral entry of SARS-CoV-2 (Niu et al., 2020; Chan et al., 2020). Luteolin, kaempferol, quercetin, apigenin, rutin, caffeic acid, chlorogenic acid, lonicerin (Xu et al., 2019). Chlorogenic acid in Flos Lonicerae Japonicae has antiviral activity against influenza A (H1N1/H3N2) and inhibition of neuraminidase (Ding et al., 2017). Homosecoiridoid alkaloids in Flos Lonicerae Japonicae have antiviral activity against the influenza virus H3N2 (Yu et al., 2013).

	Lian Qiao (Fructus Forsythiae)	Fructus Forsythiae could act on the S-protein binding site of ACE2 to block viral entry of SARS-CoV-2 (Niu et al., 2020; Chan et al., 2020). Forsythoside A has antiviral effects against influenza (Law et al., 2017). Fructus Forsythiae contains luteolin, quercetin, kaempferol, rutin, baicalin, wogonin. Lignans (forsythin) triterpenoids (betulinic acid, oleanolic acid, ursolic acid) (Dong et al., 2017).
	Huang Qin (Scutellaria Baicalensis)	Baicalin may bind to the ACE2 enzyme to block entry of SARS-CoV-2 (Chen & Du, 2020). Scutellarin is predicted to bind to the ACE2 receptor to prevent SARS-CoV-2 entry (Chen & Du, 2020). Chrysin may inhibit 3CL[pro] and baicalin may inhibit PL[pro] (Wu et al., 2020).

		Scutellarein inhibits the helicase protein of SARS-CoV-1 (Yu et al., 2012). Baicalin, chrysin, wogonin, and oroxylin A have therapeutic efficacy against acute lung injury caused by influenza A virus (H1N1) (Zhi et al., 2019). Scutellarin suppresses NLP3 inflammasome activation in macrophages, decreases NFKB, IL-6, TNF-α, and IL-1β (Liu et al., 2018; Wang et al., 2016; Tan et al., 2009). Scutellarin also protects against LPS induced acute lung injury via inhibition of NFKB activation in mice (Tan et al., 2009).
	Gan Cao (Radix Glycyrrhizae)	Glycyrrhiza Glabra contains the antiviral triterpenoid saponin, glycyrrhizin, found to inhibit SARS-CoV-1 (Cinatl et al., 2003).

		Glycyrrhizin is predicted to bind to the ACE2 receptor to prevent SARS-CoV-2 entry (Chen & Du, 2020). Glycyrrhizin inhibits IL-6 in macrophages (Liu et al., 2014). Isoliquiritigenin inhibits NFKB activation to suppress the inflammatory response in ARDS (Lago et al., 2014).
	Da Huang (Rheum Palmatum)	Emodin markedly inhibited the interaction of SARS-CoV-1 S-protein and ACE2 (Ho et al., 2007). Emodin from genus Rheum Palmatum (Da Huang) blocks 3CL[pro] (Luo et al., 2009) Emodin inhibits the 3a (viral) ion channel of SARS-CoV-1 and may potentially prevent viral release from infected cells (Schwarz et al., 2011; Schwarz et al., 2014).

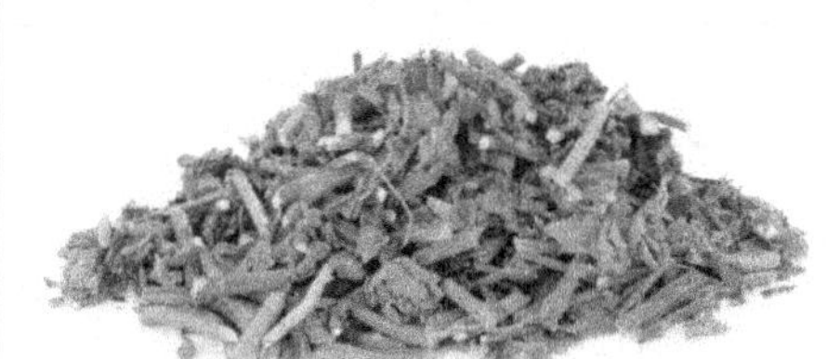	Huo Xiang (Giant Hyssop, Agastaches)	Patchouli alcohol in Guang Huo Xiang (Herba Pogostemonis) acts on the ACE2 receptor to prevent viral entry (Wu et al., 2020). Patchouli alcohol contained in Guang Huo Xiang (Herba Pogostemonis) also inhibits 3CL^{pro} and, therefore, viral replication of SARS-CoV-2 (Wu et al., 2020). Huo Xiang (Herba Pogostemonis) contains pachypodol, a tri-O-methyl ether of quercetin that inhibits several human pathogenic RNA viruses, including rhinovirus, coxsackievirus and poliovirus, acting on viral plus-strand RNA replication (Ishitsuka et al., 1982).

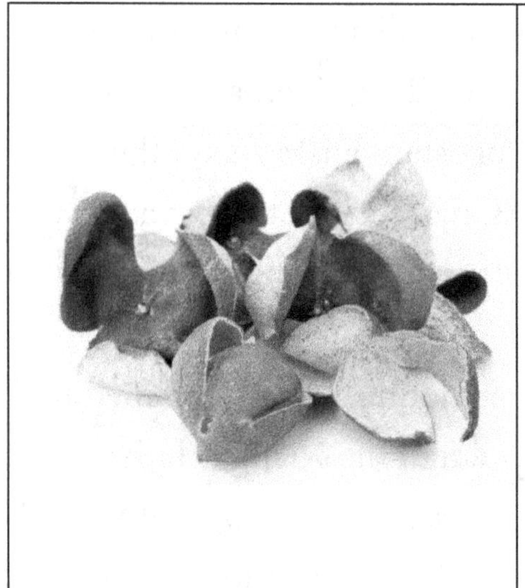	Chen Pi (Pericarpium Citri Reticulatae)	Hesperetin from Pericarpium Citri Reticulatae is predicted to bind with ACE2 (Chen & Du, 2020). Nobiletin ameliorates inflammation in acute lung injury by suppression of NFKB pathway in vivo and vitro (Li et al., 2018).

2. 3CL[pro]/M[pro]inhibition

3CL[pro] is an important CoV enzyme that plays an essential role in mediating viral replication and transcription (Jin et al., 2020). 3CL[pro] is individually responsible for releasing critical replicative enzymes such as RdRp and helicase from polyprotein precursors (Thiel et al., 2011). The main protease M[pro] of SARS-CoV-2 is also known as 3CL[pro]. Because 3- chymotrypsin-like cysteine protease (3CL[pro]) is so crucial for viral replication, it was considered as a drug target for the development of therapeutics agents for SARS-CoV-1 (Grum-Tokars et al., 2008) and is now being considered for SARS-CoV-2 (Wu et al., 2020; Zhang et al., 2020; Khaerunnisa et al., 2020).

The most studied compounds that inhibited the proteolytic activity of 3CL[pro]/M[pro] of SARS-CoV-1 are being tested as candidates for 3CL[pro] inhibition of SARS-CoV-2. These bioactive compounds include quercetin, quercetrin, cinanserin, TSL, kaempferol, sinigrin, β-sitosterol, indigo, patchouli alcohol, hesperidin, neohesperidin, chrysin, 2β-hydroxy-3,4-seco-friedelolactone-27-oic acid, isodecortinol, and cerevisterol, and andrographolide (Lau et al., 2008; Chen et al., 2008; Zhang et al., 2020; Wu et al., 2020; Khaerunnisa et al., 2020; Lin et al., 2015). This research suggests that the herbs containing these compounds may also be useful for 3CL[pro] inhibition of SARS-CoV-2.

The herbs that contain these compounds include Yu Xing Cao (Houttuynia Cordata), Xiang Chun Ye (Toona Sinensis Roem), Mian Ma Guan Zhong (Dryopteris Crassirhizoma), Ban Lan Gen (Isatis Indigotica), Huo Xiang (Herba Agastaches Pogostemonis), Zhi Shi (Fructus Aurantii Immaturus, Huang Qin (Scutellaria Baicalensis), Viola Diffusa (Zi Hua Di Ding), and Chuan Xin Lian (Andrographis Paniculata).

The following chart lists the herbs and compounds in *San Da Jie Du Tang* that might inhibit the proteolytic activity of 3CL[pro]/M[pro] of SARS-CoV-2. Please note additional studies for each herb referenced in the chart below.

Compounds in San Da Jie Tang That Might Inhibit 3CLpro/Mpro of SARS-CoV-2		
Ingredients	**Herb Name**	**Bioactive Compounds and Actions**
	Huang Qin (Scutellaria Baicalensis)	Chrysin may inhibit $3CL^{pro}$ and baicalin may inhibit PL^{pro} (Wu et al., 2020). Baicalin, chrysin, wogonin, and oroxylin A have therapeutic efficacy against acute lung injury caused by influenza A virus (H1N1) (Zhi et al., 2019). Baicalin may bind to the ACE2 enzyme to block entry of SARS-CoV-2 (Chen & Du, 2020). Scutellarein inhibits the helicase protein of SARS-CoV-1 (Yu et al., 2012). Scutellarin is predicted to bind to the ACE2 receptor to prevent SARS-CoV-2 entry (Chen & Du, 2020).

		Scutellarin suppresses NLP3 inflammasome activation in macrophages, decreases NFKB, IL-6, TNF-α, and IL-1β (Liu et al., 2018; Wang et al., 2016; Tan et al., 2009). Scutellarin also protects against LPS induced acute lung injury via inhibition of NFKB activation in mice (Tan et al., 2009).
	Yu Xing Cao (Houttuynia Cordata)	Quercetin, quercetrin, and cinanserin from the water extract of Houttuynia Cordata (Yu Xing Cao) inhibits SARS-CoV-1 3CL^{pro} (Lau et al., 2008). Houttuynia Cordata (Yu Xing Cao) blocked viral RNA-dependent RNA polymerase activity of SARS-CoV-1 (Lau et al., 2008). Plant polysaccharides from Houttuynia Cordata (Yu Xing Cao) were shown to reduce pulmonary edema,

		protein exudation, and the deposition of complement activation products, thereby mitigating acute lung injury in rats (Lu et al., 2018).
	Ban Lan Gen (Isatis Indigotica)	Sinigrin, β-sitosterol, and indigo dose-dependently inhibited cleavage activities of the 3CL^{pro} (Lin et al., 2015). Phaitanthrin D and 2,2-di (3-indolyl)-3-indolone from *Isatis Indigotica* (Ban Lan Gen) may inhibit PL^{pro} (Wu et al., 2020).
	Toona Sinensis Roem (Xiang Chun Ye)	Quercetin demonstrates potential for M^{pro} inhibition of SARS-CoV-2 (Khaerunnisa et al., 2020). TSL-1 extracted from Toona Sinensis Roem (Xiang Chun Ye) inhibits replication of SARS-CoV-1 (Chen et al., 2008).

		Toona Sinensis Roem (Xiang Chun Ye) contains quercetin, gallic acid, kaempferol, rutin, catechin, epicatechin, β-sitosterol, toosendanin, and phytol (Chia et al., 2007).
	Da Huang (Rheum Palmatum)	Emodin from genus Rheum Palmatum (Da Huang) blocks 3CL^{pro} (Luo et al., 2009) and markedly inhibited the interaction of SARS-CoV-1 S-protein and ACE2 (Ho et al., 2007). Emodin inhibits the 3a (viral) ion channel of SARS-CoV-1 and may potentially prevent viral release from infected cells (Schwarz et al., 2011; Schwarz et al., 2014).
	Huo Xiang (Giant Hyssop, Agastaches)	Patchouli alcohol contained in Guang Huo Xiang (Herba Pogostemonis) inhibits 3CL^{pro} and, therefore, viral replication of SARS-CoV-2 (Wu et al., 2020).

		Patchouli alcohol in Guang Huo Xiang (Herba Pogostemonis) also acts on the ACE2 receptor to prevent viral entry (Wu et al., 2020). Contains pachypodol, a tri-O-methyl ether of quercetin that inhibits several human pathogenic RNA viruses, including rhinovirus, coxsackievirus and poliovirus, acting on viral plus-strand RNA replication (Ishitsuka et al., 1982).
	Mian Ma Guan Zhong (Dryopteris Crassirhizoma)	Mian Ma Guan Zhong contains kaempferol, which blocks 3CL^{pro}and PL^{pro} and has the potential to inhibit SARS-CoV-2 (Zhang et al., 2020).
	Zhi Shi (Fructus Aurantii Immaturus)	Hesperidin and neohesperidin demonstrate potential as M^{pro} inhibitors (Khaerunnisa et al., 2020). Hesperetin is predicted to bind to the ACE2 receptor to

		prevent SARS-CoV-2 entry (Chen & Du, 2020). Hesperidin has high binding affinity to the helicase protein of SARS-CoV-2 (Wu et al., 2020). Fructus Aurantii Immaturus contains hesperidin, neohesperidin, hesperetin, rutin, rhoifolin, naringin (Bai et al., 2018). Hesperidin ameliorates acute lung injury (ALI) by inhibiting HMGB1 release (Liu et al., 2015). Naringin has a protective effect against ALI (Fouad et al., 2016).
	Jie Geng (Radix Platycodi)	Platycodin D demonstrated high binding affinity to PL^{pro} (Wu et al., 2020). Saponin, platycodin D, attenuates acute lung injury

		by suppressing apoptosis and inflammation in vivo and in vitro (Tao et al., 2015).
	Andrographis Paniculata (Chuan Xin Lian)	Andrographolide is predicted to inhibit 3CL[pro] and helicase proteins of SARS-CoV-2 (Wu et al., 2020). Andrographis Paniculata contains andrographolide, neoandrographolide, apigenin, luteolin (Rafi et al., 2020).
	Viola Diffusa (Zi Hua Di Ding)	2β-hydroxy-3,4-seco-friedelolactone-27-oic acid, isodecortinol, and cerevisterol from Viola Diffusa demonstrate potential as 3CL[pro] inhibitors (Wu et al., 2020). Viola Diffusa contains luteolin, quercetin, anthocyanin.

3. PL^pro inhibition

Virtual screening and computer modeling studies have revealed many naturally derived compounds with the highest binding affinity to papain-like protease (PL^pro) of SARS-CoV-2. Some of these compounds include platycodin D, baicalin, phaitanthrin D, 2,2-di (3-indolyl)-3-indolone, and kaempferol (Wu et al., 2020; Zhang et al., 2020). All of these compounds demonstrated a high binding affinity to PL^pro, suggesting the potential utility of these compounds to inhibit PL^pro of SARS-CoV-2.

The specific herbs in *San Da Jie Du Tang* that contain these compounds include Radix Platycodi (Jie Geng), Scutellaria Baicalensis (Huang Qin), Isatis Indigotica (Ban Lan Gen), and Mian Ma Guan Zhong (Dryopteris Crassirhizoma).

The following chart lists the herbs and compounds in *San Da Jie Du Tang* that might inhibit PL^pro of SARS-CoV-2. Please note additional studies for each herb referenced in the chart below.

Compounds in San Da Jie Tang That Might Inhibit PLpro of SARS-CoV-2		
Ingredients	Herb Name	Bioactive Compounds and Actions
	Huang Qin (Scutellaria Baicalensis)	Baicalin may inhibit PL^{pro} and chrysin may inhibit $3CL^{pro}$ of SARS-CoV-2 (Wu et al., 2020). Baicalin may have strong binding to the ACE2 enzyme of SARS-CoV-2 (Chen & Du, 2020). Scutellarein inhibits the helicase protein of SARS-CoV-1 (Yu et al., 2012). Scutellarin is predicted to bind to the ACE2 receptor to prevent SARS-CoV-2 entry (Chen & Du, 2020). Scutellarin suppresses NLP3 inflammasome activation in macrophages,

		decreases NFKB, IL-6, TNF-α, and IL-1β (Liu et al., 2018; Wang et al., 2016; Tan et al., 2009). Scutellarin also protects against LPS induced acute lung injury via inhibition of NFKB activation in mice (Tan et al., 2009). Baicalin, chrysin, wogonin, and oroxylin A have therapeutic efficacy against acute lung injury caused by influenza A virus (H1N1) (Zhi et al., 2019).
	Ban Lan Gen (Isatis Indigotica)	Phaitanthrin D and 2,2-di (3-indolyl)-3-indolone from Isatis Indigotica (Ban Lan Gen) may inhibit PL^{pro} (Wu et al., 2020). Sinigrin, β-sitosterol, and indigo dose-dependently inhibited cleavage activities of the 3CL^{pro} (Lin et al.,

		2015).
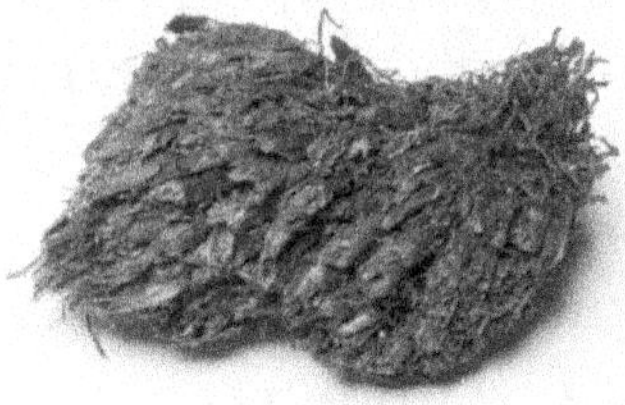	Mian Ma Guan Zhong (Dryopteris Crassirhizoma)	Mian Ma Guan Zhong contains kaempferol, which blocks PL^{pro} and 3CL^{pro}, and has the potential to inhibit SARS-CoV-2 (Zhang et al., 2020).
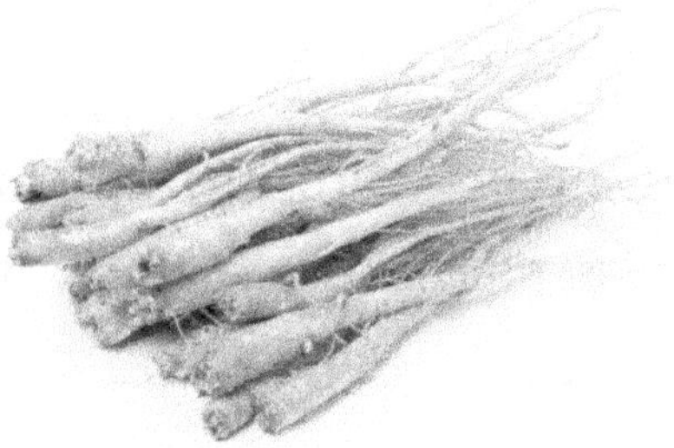	Jie Geng (Radix Platycodi)	Platycodin D demonstrated high binding affinity to PL^{pro} (Wu et al., 2020). Saponin, platycodin D, attenuates acute lung injury by suppressing apoptosis and inflammation in vivo and in vitro (Tao et al., 2015).

4. Spike Protein Binding

Binding with the surface spike (S2) protein to block the SARS-CoV-2 from entering host cells is another valuable target for the development of antiviral drugs (Wu et al., 2020). The most promising compounds that have been shown to bind with the surface spike (S2) protein of SARS-CoV-1 have included Tetra-O-galloyl-β-D-glucose (TGG) from Galla Chinensis (Wu Bei Zi) and luteolin extracted from many Chinese herbs (Yi et al., 2004). Given the homology of SARS-CoV-1 and SARS-CoV-2, these same compounds may bind with the surface spike (S2) protein of SARS-CoV-2.

The herbs in *San Da Jie Du Tang* that contain luteolin include Folium Mori (Sang Ye), Flos Lonicerae Japonicae (Jin Yin Hua), Xiang Ru (Herba Moslae), and Zi Hua Di Ding (Viola Diffusa), Lian Qiao (Fructus Forsythiae), and Chuan Xin Lian (Andrographis Paniculata). Galla Chinensis (Wu Bei Zi) contains TGG. The following chart lists the herbs and compounds that might bind with the spike protein of SARS-CoV-2.

Compounds in San Da Jie Tang That Might Bind With the Spike Protein of SARS-CoV-2		
Ingredients	**Herb Name**	**Bioactive Compounds and Actions**
	Wu Bei Zi (Galla Chinensis)	Tetra-O-galloyl-β-D-glucose (TGG) from Galla Chinensis (Wu Bei Zi) has been shown to bind with the surface spike (S2) protein of SARS-CoV-1 to block entry into the host cell (Yi et al., 2004).
	Jin Yin Hua (Flos Lonicerae Japonicae) Folium Mori (Sang Ye) Zi Hua Di Ding (Viola Diffusa), Lian Qiao (Fructus Forsythiae)	Luteolin extracted from many Chinese herbs has been shown to bind with the surface spike (S2) protein of SARS-CoV-1 to block entry into the host cell (Yi et al., 2004).

	Chuan Xin Lian (Andrographis Paniculata) Xiang Ru (Herba Moslae)	

5. Helicase Inhibition

The helicase enzyme is also involved in viral replication and therefore considered a target for anti-HCoV (human coronavirus) agents. An in vitro study by Yu et al. (2012) reported that scutellarein potently inhibited the nsP13 (SARS-CoV-1 helicase protein) in vitro by affecting ATPase activity. Recent virtual screening studies of anti-SARS-CoV-2 compounds revealed that hesperidin has a high binding affinity to the helicase protein (Wu et al., 2020).

This research suggests that the following herbs containing these compounds may also lead to helicase inhibition of SARS-CoV-2. The following chart lists the compounds in *San Da Jie Du Tang* that may inhibit the helicase protein of SARS-CoV-2. Please note additional studies for each herb referenced in the chart below.

Compounds in San Da Jie Du Tang That Might Inhibit the Helicase Protein of SARS-CoV-2		
Ingredients	**Herb Name**	**Bioactive Compounds and Actions**
	Huang Qin (Scutellaria Baicalensis)	Scutellarein inhibits the helicase protein of SARS-CoV-1 (Yu et al., 2012). Baicalin may have strong binding to the ACE2 enzyme of SARS-CoV-2 (Chen & Du, 2020). Chrysin may inhibit $3CL^{pro}$ and baicalin may inhibit PL^{pro} (Wu et al., 2020). Scutellarin is predicted to bind to the ACE2 receptor to prevent SARS-CoV-2 entry (Chen & Du, 2020). Scutellarin suppresses NLP3 inflammasome activation in macrophages, decreases NFKB, IL-6, TNF-α, and IL-1β (Liu et

		al., 2018; Wang et al., 2016; Tan et al., 2009). Scutellarin also protects against LPS induced acute lung injury via inhibition of NFKB activation in mice (Tan et al., 2009). Baicalin, chrysin, wogonin, and oroxylin A have therapeutic efficacy against acute lung injury caused by influenza A virus (H1N1) (Zhi et al., 2019).
	Zhi Shi (Fructus Aurantii Immaturus)	Hesperidin has high binding affinity to the helicase protein of SARS-CoV-2 (Wu et al., 2020). Hesperidin and neohesperidin demonstrate potential as M^{pro} inhibitors (Khaerunnisa et al., 2020). Hesperetin is predicted to bind to the ACE2 receptor to prevent SARS-CoV-2 entry (Chen & Du, 2020).

		Hesperidin ameliorates acute lung injury (ALI) by inhibiting HMGB1 release (Liu et al., 2015). Fructus Aurantii Immaturus contains hesperidin, neohesperidin, hesperetin, rutin, rhoifolin, naringin (Bai et al., 2018). Naringin has a protective effect against ALI (Fouad et al., 2016).

6. RNA- dependent RNA polymerase (RdRp) inhibition

RNA-dependent RNA polymerase (RdRp) is an enzyme responsible for RNA synthesis and another potential target of SARS-CoV-2 as it was for SARS-CoV-1. RdRp is the target of the antiviral drug Remdesivir. One of the herbs in *San Da Jie Du Tang*, Houttuynia Cordata (Yu Xing Cao), has been shown to inhibit RNA-dependent RNA polymerase activity of SARS-CoV-1 (Lau et al., 2008). The research suggests that Houttuynia Cordata (Yu Xing Cao) may also inhibit RNA-dependent RNA polymerase activity of SARS-CoV-2. The following chart lists the compounds in *San Da Jie Du Tang* that might inhibit the RNA-dependent RNA polymerase of SARS-CoV-2. Please note additional studies for each herb referenced in the chart below.

Compounds in San Da Jie Du Tang That Might Inhibit RNA-dependent RNA Polymerase		
Ingredients	Herb Name	Bioactive Compounds and Actions
	Yu Xing Cao (Houttuynia Cordata)	Houttuynia Cordata (Yu Xing Cao) blocked viral RNA-dependent RNA polymerase activity of SARS-CoV-1 (Lau et al., 2008). Quercetin, quercetrin, and cinanserin from the water extract of Houttuynia Cordata (Yu Xing Cao) inhibits SARS-CoV-1 3CLpro (Lau et al., 2008). Plant polysaccharides from Houttuynia Cordata (Yu Xing Cao) were shown to reduce pulmonary edema, protein exudation, and the deposition of complement activation products, thereby mitigating acute lung injury in rats (Lu et al., 2018).

7. Viroporin 3a ion channel inhibition

Activation of the 3a (viral) ion channels is involved in the production and release of SARS-CoV-1 (Lu et al., 2006). Emodin is one of the natural compounds that has been shown to inhibit the 3a (viral) ion channel of SARS-CoV-1 and could potentially prevent viral release from infected cells (Schwarz et al., 2011; Schwarz et al., 2014). The research suggests that emodin and the herbs that contain it, such as Da Huang (Rheum Palmatum), may also inhibit the 3a ion channels of SARS-CoV-2.

The following chart lists the compounds in *San Da Jie Du Tang* that may inhibit the Viroporin 3a ion channel. Please note additional studies referenced in the chart below.

Compounds in San Da Jie Du Tang That Might Inhibit the Viroporin 3a ion channel		
Ingredients	**Herb Name**	**Bioactive Compounds and Actions**
	Da Huang (Rheum Palmatum)	Emodin inhibits the 3a ion channel of SARS-CoV-1 and may potentially prevent viral release from infected cells (Schwarz et al., 2011; Schwarz et al., 2014). Emodin from genus Rheum Palmatum (Da Huang) blocks

		3CL^{pro} (Luo et al., 2009) and markedly inhibited the interaction of SARS-CoV-1 S-protein and ACE2 (Ho et al., 2007).

8. TMPRSS2 Inhibition

The type-II transmembrane serine protease (TMPRSS2) enzyme is also considered a possible target for antiviral drug discovery for SARS-CoV-2. In a recent virtual screening study, Wu et al. (2020) found that compounds in *San Da Jie Du Tang*, such as neoandrographolide in Andrographis Paniculata (Chuan Xin Lian), demonstrated potential for TMPRSS2 inhibition. The following chart lists the compounds included in *San Da Jie Du Tang* that might inhibit the TMPRSS2 enzyme of SARS-CoV-2. Please note additional studies referenced in the chart below.

Compounds in San Da Jie Du Tang That Might Inhibit TMPRSS2		
	Andrographis Paniculata (Chuan Xin Lian)	Neoandrographolide in Andrographis Paniculata (Chuan Xin Lian) demonstrated potential for TMPRSS2 inhibition (Wu et al., 2020).

		Andrographolide is predicted to inhibit 3CL[pro] and helicase proteins of SARS-CoV-2 (Wu et al., 2020). Andrographis Paniculata contains andrographolide, neoandrographolide, apigenin, luteolin (Rafi et al., 2020).

The following chart summarizes all of the herbs and compounds in *San Da Jie Du Tang* that might inhibit SARS-CoV-2 at all levels to block viral entry and replication.

Summary of Herbs and Compounds in San Da Jie Du Tang That Might Inhibit SARS-CoV-2		
ACE2 blockade	Glycyrrhizin	Gan Cao (Radix Glycyrrhizae)
	Scutellarin	Huang Qin (Scutellaria Baicalensis)
	Hesperetin	Chen Pi (Pericarpium Citri Reticulatae)
	Emodin	Da Huang (Rheum

		Palmatum)
	Chlorogenic Acid	Jin Yin Hua (Flos Lonicerae Japonicae)
	Forsythoside A	Lian Qiao (Fructus Forsythiae)
	Patchouli alcohol	Huo Xiang (Herba Agastaches Pogostemonis)
$3CL^{pro}/M^{pro}$ inhibition	Quercetin, quercetrin, and cinanserin	Yu Xing Cao (Houttuynia Cordata)
	Quercetin and TSL	Xiang Chun Ye (Toona Sinensis Roem)
	Kaempferol	Mian Ma Guan Zhong (Dryopteris Crassirhizoma)
	Sinigrin, β-sitosterol, and indigo	Ban Lan Gen (Isatis Indigotica)
	Patchouli alcohol	Huo Xiang (Herba Agastaches Pogostemonis)
	Hesperidin and Neohesperidin	Zhi Shi (Fructus Aurantii Immaturus)

	Chrysin	Huang Qin (Scutellaria Baicalensis)
	Andrographolide	Chuan Xin Lian (Andrographis Paniculata)
	2β-hydroxy-3,4-seco-friedelolactone-27-oic acid, isodecortinol, and cerevisterol	Zi Hua Di Ding (Viola Diffusa)
PL^{pro} inhibition	Platycodin D	Jie Geng (Radix Platycodi)
	Baicalin	Huang Qin (Scutellaria Baicalensis)
	Phaitanthrin D and 2,2-di (3-indolyl)-3-indolone	Ban Lan Gen (Isatis Indigotica)
	Kaempferol	Mian Ma Guan Zhong (Dryopteris Crassirhizoma)
Spike protein binding	Tetra-O-galloyl-β-D-glucose (TGG)	Wu Bei Zi (Galla Chinensis)
	Luteolin	Sang Ye (Folium Mori), Jin Yin Hua (Flos Lonicerae Japonicae), Xiang Ru

		(Herba Moslae), Zi Hua Di Ding (Viola Diffusa), Lian Qiao (Fructus Forsythiae), and Chuan Xin Lian (Andrographis Paniculata)
Helicase inhibition	Scutellarein Hesperidin	Huang Qin (Scutellaria Baicalensis) Zhi Shi (Fructus Aurantii Immaturus)
RNA- dependent RNA polymerase (RdRp) inhibition	Quercetin, quercetrin, and cinanserin	Yu Xing Cao (Houttuynia Cordata)
Viroporin 3a ion channel inhibition	Emodin	Da Huang (Rheum Palmatum)
TMPRSS2 inhibition	Neoandrographolide	Chuan Xin Lian (Andrographis Paniculata)

Below is a summary chart of herbs (TCM and botanical names) in *San Da Jie Du Tang* that may inhibit SARS-CoV-2.

Herbs in San Da Jie Du Tang That May Inhibit SARS-CoV-2	
ACE2 blockade	Gan Cao (Radix Glycyrrhizae)
	Huang Qin (Scutellaria Baicalensis)
	Chen Pi (Pericarpium Citri Reticulatae)
	Da Huang (Rheum Palmatum)
	Jin Yin Hua (Flos Lonicerae Japonicae)
	Lian Qiao (Fructus Forsythiae)
	Huo Xiang (Herba Agastaches Pogostemonis)
3CL^{pro}/M^{pro} inhibition	Yu Xing Cao (Houttuynia Cordata)
	Xiang Chun Ye (Toona Sinensis Roem)
	Mian Ma Guan Zhong (Dryopteris Crassirhizoma)
	Ban Lan Gen (Isatis Indigotica)
	Huo Xiang (Herba Agastaches Pogostemonis)
	Zhi Shi (Fructus Aurantii Immaturus)
	Huang Qin (Scutellaria Baicalensis)
	Chuan Xin Lian (Andrographis Paniculata)
PL^{pro} inhibition	Jie Geng (Radix Platycodi)
	Huang Qin (Scutellaria Baicalensis)
	Ban Lan Gen (Isatis Indigotica)
	Mian Ma Guan Zhong (Dryopteris Crassirhizoma)
Spike protein binding	Wu Bei Zi (Galla Chinensis)
	Jin Yin Hua (Flos Lonicerae Japonicae)
	Xiang Ru (Herba Moslae)
	Zi Hua Di Ding (Viola Diffusa)
	Lian Qiao (Fructus Forsythiae)

	Chuan Xin Lian (Andrographis Paniculata)
Helicase inhibition	Huang Qin (Scutellaria Baicalensis) Zhi Shi (Fructus Aurantii Immaturus
RNA- dependent RNA polymerase (RdRp) inhibition	Yu Xing Cao (Houttuynia Cordata)
Viroporin 3a ion channel inhibition	Da Huang (Rheum Palmatum)
TMPRSS2 inhibition	Chuan Xin Lian (Andrographis Paniculata)

Below is an additional summary chart of herbs (pin yin only) in *San Da Jie Du Tang* that may inhibit SARS-CoV-2.

Herbs in San Da Jie Du Tang That May Inhibit SARS-CoV-2	
ACE2 blockade	Gan Cao Huang Qin Chen Pi Da Huang Jin Yin Hua Lian Qiao Huo Xiang
3CL^{pro}/M^{pro}inhibition	Yu Xing Cao Xiang Chun Ye Mian Ma Guan Zhong Ban Lan Gen

	Huo Xiang
	Zhi Shi
	Huang Qin
	Chuan Xin Lian
PL^{pro} inhibition	Jie Geng
	Huang Qin
	Ban Lan Gen
	Mian Ma Guan Zhong
Spike protein binding	Wu Bei Zi
	Jin Yin Hua
	Xiang Ru
	Zi Hua Di Ding
	Lian Qiao
	Chuan Xin Lian
Helicase inhibition	Huang Qin
	Zhi Shi
RNA- dependent RNA polymerase (RdRp) inhibition	Yu Xing Cao
Viroporin 3a ion channel inhibition	Da Huang
TMPRSS2 inhibition	Chuan Xin Lian

Herbs for Respiratory Support in San Da Jie Du Tang

While almost all of the herbs in *San Da Jie Du Tang* have been used traditionally for viral respiratory illnesses, some of the herbs have multiple compounds that make them excellent candidates for the current pandemic. For example, Huang Qin (Scutellaria Baicalensis) contains baicalin, which is not only predicted to bind to the ACE2 receptor to block entry of SARS-CoV-2 (Chen & Du, 2020) but may also inhibit PL^{pro} (Wu et al., 2020).

Huang Qin (Scutellaria Baicalensis) also contains chrysin, which may inhibit 3CL^{pro} and scutellarein, which inhibits the helicase protein of SARS-CoV-1 (Yu et al., 2012). Baicalin, chrysin, wogonin, and oroxylin A have demonstrated therapeutic efficacy against acute lung injury caused by the influenza A virus (H1N1) (Zhi et al., 2019). Huang Qin (Scutellaria Baicalensis) also contains scutellarin, which suppresses NLP3 inflammasome activation in macrophages and decreases NFKB, IL-6, TNF-α and IL-1β (Liu et al., 2018; Wang et al., 2016; Tan et al., 2009). Scutellarin also protects against LPS induced acute lung injury via inhibition of NFKB activation in mice (Tan et al., 2009).

Jin Yin Hua (Flos Lonicerae Japonicae), used historically for respiratory infection, contains many bioactive compounds including luteolin, kaempferol, quercetin, apigenin, rutin, caffeic acid, chlorogenic acid, and lonicerin (Xu et al., 2019). Chlorogenic acid in Jin Yin Hua (Flos Lonicerae Japonicae has antiviral activity against influenza A (H1N1/H3N2) and inhibition of neuraminidase (Ding et al., 2017). Homosecoiridoid alkaloids in Flos Lonicerae Japonicae (Jin Yin Hua) have antiviral activity against the influenza virus H3N2 (Yu et al., 2013). Notably, Jin Yin Hua (Flos Lonicerae Japonicae), is predicted to act on the S-protein binding site of the ACE2 receptor to block viral entry of SARS-CoV-2 (Niu et al., 2020; Chan et al., 2020).

Lian Qiao (Fructus Forsythiae), another herb used for respiratory illnesses, contains luteolin, quercetin, kaempferol, rutin, baicalin, forsythoside A, wogonin as well as lignans (forsythin), and triterpenoids (betulinic acid, oleanolic acid, ursolic acid) (Law et al., 2017; Dong et al., 2017). Forsythoside A has antiviral effects against influenza (Law et al., 2017). Lian Qiao (Fructus Forsythiae) was also predicted to act on the S-protein binding site of ACE2 to block viral entry of SARS-CoV-2 (Niu et al., 2020; Chan et al., 2020).

Jie Geng (Radix Platycodi) has been used for respiratory illnesses for hundreds of years. Jie Geng (Radix Platycodi) contains platycodin D, which demonstrated not only high binding affinity to PL^{pro} (Wu et al., 2020), but also attenuates acute lung injury by suppressing apoptosis and inflammation in vivo and in vitro (Tao et al., 2015).

Sang Ye, has traditionally been used for respiratory illnesses and contains many potent compounds, including rutin, isoquercitrin, astragalin, kaempferol, quercetin, chlorogenic acid, morin, and gallic acid, all known for their antiviral and anti-inflammatory effects (Zhang et al., 2017; Chen et al., 2018; Kim et al., 2014).

Herba Moslae (Xiang Ru) is useful for viral respiratory infections and contains many similar flavonoids as Herba Ephedrae (Ma Huang), including luteolin, quercetin, and apigenin (Hu et al., 2010).

Bo He (Herba Menthae Haplocalyx) contains diosmin, which downregulates T cell receptors, proinflammatory cytokines, and NFKB activation against LPS-induced acute lung injury in mice (Imam et al., 2015). Bo He (Herba Menthae Haplocalyx) also contains quercetin, hesperetin, and hesperidin, which have been shown to act on 3CL[pro] (quercetin, hesperidin), ACE2 (hesperetin), and the helicase protein (hesperidin) (Lau et al., 2008; Chen and Du 2020; Wu et al., 2020).

Ku Xing Ren (Semen Armeniacae Amarum) contains amygdalin, has been shown to inhibit NFKB and NLRP3 signaling pathways in LPS-induced acute lung injury (Zhang et al., 2017). Amygdalin also has an antitussive effect (Miyagoshi et al., 1986).

Zhi Shi (Fructus Aurantii Immaturus) contains hesperidin, neohesperidin, hesperetin, rutin, rhoifolin, naringin (Bai et al., 2018). Naringin has been shown to have a protective effect against acute lung injury (ALI) (Fouad et al., 2016). Notably, hesperidin and neohesperidin both demonstrate potential as M^{pro} inhibitors (Khaerunnisa et al., 2020). Hesperidin also has a high binding affinity to the helicase protein of SARS-CoV-2 (Wu et al., 2020), and ameliorates acute lung injury (ALI) by inhibiting HMGB1 release (Liu et al., 2015). Hesperetin is predicted to bind to the ACE2 receptor to prevent SARS-CoV-2 entry (Chen & Du, 2020).

Finally, Gan Cao (Glycyrrhiza Glabra) contains the antiviral triterpenoid saponin, glycyrrhizin, found to inhibit SARS-CoV-1 (Cinatl et al., 2003). Notably, Glycyrrhizin is also predicted to bind to the ACE2 receptor to prevent SARS-CoV-2 entry (Chen & Du, 2020). Glycyrrhizin has also been shown to inhibit IL-6 in LPS-induced cytokines expression in macrophage (Liu et al., 2014). Also, the compound isoliquiritigenin, in Gan Cao (Glycyrrhiza Glabra), inhibits NFKB activation to suppress the inflammatory response in ARDS (Lago et al., 2014).

Safety of Medicinal Herbs

Now that we have explored the potential benefits of *San Da Jie Du Tang*, we need to consider the safety of medicinal herbs. Herbs are generally recognized as safe, but there are some precautions. For example, the herb Dryopteris Crassirhizoma (Guan Zhong) is considered to be slightly toxic and needs to be used with caution (Dharmananda, 2003).

It is important to remember that herbs such as Chuan Xin Lian (Andrographis Paniculata) may increase immune cells that may already get overexpressed in autoimmune disease patients. Therefore practitioners and herb companies should caution the use and promotion of Chuan Xin Lian (Andrographis Paniculata) for patients with autoimmune diseases. An alternate formula without Chuan Xin Lian (Andrographis Paniculata) may be another option.
Also, some compounds such as baicalin in Huang Qin (Scutellaria Baicalensis) may magnify or oppose the effect of pharmaceuticals and should be carefully evaluated for those on medications (Tian et al., 2013; Fong et al., 2015). Practitioners and herb companies are also encouraged to check for and list hidden allergens in the formulas for those with food allergies or sensitivities to ingredients such as Ku Xing Ren (Semen Armeniacae Amarum).

Final Thoughts

As the pandemic continues to spread out of control, especially in the United States, novel solutions are urgently needed. The herbs reviewed in this guide represent a treasure trove of potent compounds for drug development. The novel formula *San Da Jie Du Tang* contains multiple compounds that may act to block viral attachment, entry, and replication. All of these compounds are potent candidates for drug development for the current pandemic.

Notably, there is an enormous amount of research on herbs in the Chinese pharmacy that may be useful for decreasing the severity of viral respiratory infections. We need an antiviral formula that can halt the progression from fever, fatigue, and dry cough to dyspnea and acute respiratory distress. *San Da Jie Du Tang* contains all of the compounds that can potentially dismantle SARS-CoV-2 at all levels and might be used at to halt the progression and damaging effects of severe viral respiratory infections.

Given the current research, it is hoped that herb companies will start creating new potent antiviral herbal formulas for the initial stages of infection. Then researchers can run a randomized controlled trial to test the efficacy of the antiviral herbal compounds in formulas such as *San Da Jie Du Tang* for patients. Until then, practitioners can study the research about the compounds in herbs used for SARS-CoV-1 and other viral respiratory infections to create the most precise formulas to halt and mitigate the severity of the pandemic. Thanks for taking the time to read this book. For more information about other books and continuing education classes for CA Licensed Acupuncturists, please visit anneangelone.com.

References

Bai, Y., Zheng, Y.J., Pang, W.J., Peng, W., Wu, H., Yao, H.L.,…Su, W.W. (2018). Identification and Comparison of Constituents of Aurantii Fructus and Aurantii Fructus Immaturus by UFLC-DAD-Triple TOF-MS/MS. *Molecules*, 23(4), 803. MDPI AG. http://dx.doi.org/10.3390/molecules23040803

Chan, K.W., Wang, V.T., & Tang, S.C.W. (2020, March). Covid-19: An Update on the Epidemiological, Clinical, Preventive and Therapeutic Evidence and Guidelines of Integrative Chinese–Western Medicine for the Management of 2019 Novel Coronavirus Disease. *The American Journal of Chinese Medicine*, Vol. 48, No. 3, 1–26.

Chen, H., & Du, Q. (2020). Potential Natural Compounds for Preventing 2019-nCoV Infection. *Preprints.org*. 2020010358.

Chen, Z., Du, X., Yang, Y., Cui, X., Zhang, Z., & Li, Y. (2018). Comparative study of chemical composition and active components against α-glucosidase of various medicinal parts of Morus alba L. *Biomedical Chromatography: BMC*, 32(11), e4328. https://doi.org/10.1002/bmc.4328

Dharmananda, S. *SARS and Chinese Medicine. (2003). How the Chinese People and Institutions Responded with Herbs.* Institute for Traditional Medicine, Portland, Oregon. http://www.itmonline.org/arts/sars.htm

Dong, Z.L., Lu, X.Y., Tong, X.L., Dong, Y.Q., Tang, L., & Li, M.H. (2017, September). Forsythiae Fructus: A Review on its Phytochemistry, Quality Control, Pharmacology and Pharmacokinetics. *Molecules*, 22(9): 1466. DOI: 10.3390/molecules22091466

Fouad, A., Albuali, W., & Jresat, I. (2016, January). Protective effect of naringenin against lipopolysaccharide-induced acute lung injury in rats. *Pharmacology*.

Khaerunnisa, S., Kurniawan, H., Awaluddin, R., Suharta, S., & Soetjipto, S. (2020, March). Potential Inhibitor of Covid-19 Main Protease (Mpro) from Several Medicinal Plant Compounds in Molecular Docking Study. *Preprints.org*. [Epub ahead of print]

Ho, T.Y., Wu, S.L., Chen, J.C., Li, C.C., & Hsiang C.Y. (2007, May). Emodin blocks the SARS-Coronavirus spike protein and angiotensin-converting enzyme 2 interaction. *Antiviral Research*, 74(2): 92–101. DOI: 10.1016/j..2006.04.014

Ho, T., Wu, S., Chen, J., Li, C., & Hsiang, C. (2007). Emodin blocks the SARS-Coronavirus spike protein and angiotensin-converting enzyme 2 interaction. *Antiviral Research*, 74:92–101.

Hu, H.W., Xie, X.M., Zhang, P.Z., & Shu, R.G. (2010). (Study on the flavonoids from Mosla chinensis 'jiangxiangru'). *Zhong yao cai = Zhongyaocai Journal of Chinese medicinal materials*, 33. 218-9.

Imam F., Al-Harbi, N.O., Al-Harbi, M.M., Ansari, M.A., Zoheir, K.M., Iqbal, M.,…Ahmad, S.F. (2015). Diosmin downregulates the expression of T cell receptors, proinflammatory cytokines and NF-κB activation against LPS-induced acute lung injury in mice. *Pharmacology Research*, 102:1–11

Ishitsuka, H., Ohsawa, C., Ohiwa, T., Umeda, I., & Suhara, Y. (1982, October) Antipicornavirus flavone Ro 09-0179. *Antimicrobial Agents and Chemotherapy*, 22(4):611-6.

Kim, D., Kang, Y.M., Jin, W.Y., Sung, Y., Choi, G., & Kim, H.K. (2014). Antioxidant activities and polyphenol content of Morus alba leaf extracts collected from varying regions. *Biomedical Reports*, 2, 675-680. https://doi.org/10.3892/br.2014.294

Lago, J.H.G., Toledo-Arruda, A.C., Mernak, M., Barrosa, K.H., Martins, M.A., Tibério L.F.L.C., & Prado C.M. (2014). Structure-Activity Association of Flavonoids in Lung Diseases. *Brazil Molecules,* 19(3), 3570-3595; https://doi.org/10.3390/molecules19033570

Lau, K.M., Lee, K.M., Koon, C.M., Cheung, C.S., Lau, C.P., Ho, H.M.,…Fung, K.P. (2008, June). Immunomodulatory and anti-SARS activities of Houttuynia Cordata. *Journal of Ethnopharmacology*, 118(1):79-85. DOI: 10.1016/j.jep.2008.03.018

Law, H.Y., Yang, L.H., Lau, S.Y., & Chan, G.C. (2017). Antiviral effect of forsythoside A from Forsythia suspensa (Thunb.) Vahl fruit against influenza A virus through reduction of viral M1 protein. *Journal of Ethnopharmacology*, 209: 236-247.

Li, W., Zhao, R., Wang, X., Liu, F., Zhao, J., Yao, Q.,…Niu, X. (2018). Nobiletin-ameliorated lipopolysaccharide-induced inflammation in acute lung injury by suppression of NF-kappaB pathway in vivo and vitro. *Inflammation*, 41 (3), pp. 996-1007.

Lin, C.W., Tsai, F.J., Tsai, C.H., Lai, C.C., Wan, L., Ho, T.Y.,…Chao, P.D. (2005, October). Anti-SARS-Coronavirus 3C-like protease effects of Isatis indigotica root and plant-derived phenolic compounds. *Antiviral Research*, 68(1):36-42.

Liu, X.X., Yu, D.D., Chen, M.J., Sun, T., Li, G., Huang, W.J.,…Ren, B.X. (2015). Hesperidin ameliorates lipopolysaccharide-induced acute lung injury in mice by inhibiting HMGB1 release. *International immunopharmacology*, 25(2), 370–376. https://doi.org/10.1016/j.intimp.2015.02.022

Liu, Y., Jing, Y.Y., & Zeng, C.Y. (2018, January). Scutellarin suppresses NLRP3 Inflammasome activation in macrophages and protects mice against bacterial sepsis. *Frontiers in Pharmacology*, 8:975. DOI:10.3389/fphar.2017.00975

Liu, Z., Zhong, J. Y., Gao, E. N., & Yang, H. (2014). Effects of glycyrrhizin acid and licorice flavonoids on LPS-induced cytokines expression in macrophage. *Zhongguo Zhong yao za zhi = Zhongguo zhongyao zazhi = China journal of Chinese Materia Medica*, 39(19), 3841–3845.

Lu, Y., Jiang, J., Ling, L.J., Zhang, Y.Y., Li, H., & Chen, D.F. (2018). Beneficial effects of Houttuynia Cordata polysaccharides on "two-hit" acute lung injury and endotoxic fever in rats associated with anti-complementary activities. *Acta Pharmaceutica Sinica B.* https://doi.org/10.1016/j.apsb.2017.11.003

Middleton, E., & Kandaswami, C. (1992). Effects of flavonoids on immune and inflammatory cell functions. *Biochemical Pharmacology*, 43, 1167–1179.

Miyagoshi, M., Amagaya, S., & Ogihara, Y. (1986) Antitussive effects of L-ephedrine, amygdalin, and makyokansekito (Chinese traditional medicine) using a cough model induced by sulfur dioxide gas in mice. *Planta Medica*, 4, 275–278.

Niu, M., Wang, R.L., Wang, Z.X., Zhang, P., Bai, Z.F., Jing, J.,... Xiao, X.H. (2020, March). Rapid establishment of traditional Chinese medicine prevention and treatment of 2019-nCoV based on clinical experience and molecular docking. *Zhongguo Zhong Yao Za Zhi*, 45(6):1213-1218. DOI: 10.19540/j.cnki.cjcmm.20200206.501.

Rafi, M., Devi, A.F., & Syafitri, U.D. (2020). Classification of Andrographis paniculata extracts by solvent extraction using HPLC fingerprint and chemometric analysis. *BMC Research Notes*, 13, 56. https://doi.org/10.1186/s13104-020-4920-x

Schwarz, S., Wang, K., Yu, W.J., Sun, B., & Schwarz, W. (2011). Emodin inhibits current through SARS-associated coronavirus 3a protein. *Antiviral Research*, 90:64-9.

Schwarz, S., Sauter, D., Wang, K., Zhang, R.H., Sun, B., Karioti, A.,…
Schwarz, W. (2014, February). Kaempferol Derivatives as antiviral drugs
against the 3a Channel Protein of Coronavirus. *Planta Medica*, 80(02-03):
177–182. DOI: 10.1055/s-0033-1360277

Tan, Z.H., Y, L.H., Wei, H.L., & Liu, G.T. (2009, September) Scutellarin
protects against lipopolysaccharide-induced acute lung injury via
inhibition of NF-κB activation in mice. *Journal of Asian Natural Products
Research*, 12:3, pp. 175- 184.
https://doi.org/10.1080/10286020903347906

Tao, W., Su, Q., Wang, H., Guo, S., Chen, Y., Duan, J., & Wang, S. (2015).
Platycodin D attenuates acute lung injury by suppressing apoptosis and
inflammation in vivo and in vitro. *International Immunopharmacology*, 27
(1) pp. 138-147.

Thiel, V., Ivanov, K.A., Putics, A., Hertzig, T., Schelle, B., Bayer,
S.,…Ziebuhr, J. (2003, September). Mechanisms and enzymes involved
in SARS coronavirus genome expression. *Journal of General Virology*,
84:2305-15.

Tian, X., Cheng, Z.Y., Jin, H., Gao, J., & Qiao, H.L. (2013). Inhibitory
Effects of Baicalin on the Expression and Activity of CYP3A Induce the
Pharmacokinetic Changes of Midazolam in Rats. *Evidence Based
Complementary and Alternative Medicine*, 179643.

Wu, C.R., Yang, L., Yang, Y.Y., Zhang, P., Zhong, W., Wang, Y.L.,…Li, H.
(2020, February) Analysis of therapeutic targets for SARS-CoV-2 and

discovery of potential drugs by computational method. *Acta Pharmaceutica Sinica B.* https://doi.org/10.1016/j.apsb.2020.02.008

Wu, Q.F., Zhu, W.R., Yan, Y.L., Zhang, X.X., Jiang, Y.Q., & Zhang, F.L. (2016). Anti-H1N1 influenza effects and its possible mechanism of Huanglian Xiangru Decoction. *Journal of ethnopharmacology*, 185, 282–288. https://doi.org/10.1016/j.jep.2016.02.042

Xu, Z.R., Kun, Li., Pan, T.W., Liu, J., Bin, Li., Li, C.X.,…Liu, X.G. (2019, July). Lonicerin, an anti-algE flavonoid against Pseudomonas aeruginosa virulence screened from Shuanghuanglian formula by molecule docking based strategy. *Journal of Ethnopharmacology*, Volume 239, 111909. https://doi.org/10.1016/j.jep.2019.111909

Yi, L., Li, Z.G., Yuan, K.H., Qu, X.X., Chen, J., Wang, G.W.,… Xia, X.J. (2004). Small molecules blocking the entry of severe acute respiratory syndrome coronavirus into host cells. *Journal of Virology*, 78:11334-9.

Yu, M.S., Lee, J., Lee, J.M., Kim, Y., Chin, Y.W. & Jee, J.G. (2012). Identification of myricetin and scutellarein as novel chemical inhibitors of the SARS-Coronavirus helicase, nsP13. *Bioorganic and Medicinal Chemistry Letters*, 22:4049-54

Zhang, A., Pan, W.Y., Lv, J., & Wu, H. (2017). Protective effect of amygdalin on LPS-induced acute lung injury by inhibiting NF-kappaB and NLRP3 signaling pathways. *Inflammation*, 40 (3) (2017), pp. 745-751.

Zhang, L.W., Ji, T., Su, S. L., Shang, E. X., Guo, S., Guo, J. M.,…Duan, J. A. (2017). Pharmacokinetics of Mori Folium Flavones and Alkaloids in

Normal and Diabetic Rats. *Zhongguo Zhong yao za zhi = Zhongguo zhongyao zazhi = China journal of Chinese materia medica*, 42(21), 4218–4225. https://doi.org/10.19540/j.cnki.cjcmm.20170901.008

Zhi, H.J., Zhu, H.Y., Zhang, Y.Y., Lu, Y., Li, H., & Chen, D.F. (2019). In vivo effect of quantified flavonoids-enriched extract of Scutellaria baicalensis root on acute lung injury induced by influenza A virus. *Phytomedicine*, 57, pp. 105-116

More books by Anne Angelone

<u>Functional Herbal Medicine and Phytonutrition</u>

<u>Functional Scalp Acupuncture</u>

<u>The Acupuncture Trip</u>

<u>The Autoimmune Diet</u>

<u>If The Buddha Had an Autoimmune Disease</u>

<u>The Autoimmune Paleo Breakthrough</u>

<u>The Paleo Autoimmune Protocol</u>

<u>The Histamine Free Paleo Breakthrough</u>

<u>The FODMAP Free Paleo Breakthrough</u>

<u>Gut Clear</u>

<u>Beyond Cannabis</u>